STOP SUGAR CRAVING FAST!
Lose Weight By Totally Ending Your Craving For Sugar.

By Gary Pickler

Lulu
2014

STOP SUGAR CRAVING FAST!
Lose Weight By Totally Ending Your Craving For Sugar.

By Gary Pickler

Lulu
2015

Stop Sugar Craving Fast! Lose Weight By Totally Ending Your Craving For Sugar.
Copyright © 2015 by Gary Pickler
ISBN13: 978-1-312-86737-6

This book is not intended as medical advice. It's intent is solely informational and educational. Please, consult a health professional if you have questions about your health. The author and publisher are not liable for any damages or negative consequences from any treatment, action, application, or preparation, to any person reading or following the information in this book.

First Printing   : 2015
Editing, page design, proof reading : Bruno Curfs
Publisher   : Lulu

Table of Contents

Introduction

My book's purpose is to *stop your sugar craving*, so that you'll be healthier, and lose weight. This brief book, of useful instruction, will do exactly that!

Two hundred more pages, of theory, philosophy, and rambling, are totally unnecessary. I've gotten right to the point, to avoid wasting your precious time!

1

Why This Book Works So Fast And So Well

It has been recently discovered[1] that eating silica-rich foods stops all craving for sugar. Silica, previously categorized as a minor trace mineral, is really *much more* than that! Silica, as a *required nutrient*, gives us an astonishing amount of needed health benefits (see chapter 4). But the bottom line is that your craving for sugar can fairly easily be stopped, by eating silica-rich foods!

Once sugar is stopped, you'll feel better, begin to be much healthier, and begin to lose unneeded weight. The longer you (easily) continue to eat no sugar, the more pounds you'll shed, until a healthier, happier, much trimmer and slimmer you, becomes a reality!

---

[1]The discovery was made in 2012, by Anthony Shkreli, and is documented (in extensive detail) in his book *You Are Not Addicted, You Are Starving*. For incredibly more detail, buy his 208 page book, and read it.

2

Why Sugar Is Bad For You, Explained In A Nutshell

Sugar (chemically) is about half glucose and half fructose. The glucose-half is OK, because it's what your body uses naturally, for energy. But the fructose-half goes straight to your liver to be processed (just as if it were a toxin or poison). After processing, uric acid exits the liver, causing (1) gout, and (2) hypertension. Fatty acids also exit the liver (after processing), causing (1) weight gain and obesity, (2) Cardiovascular Disease (Heart Attack, Stroke, Angina), (3) Liver Cirrhosis (just like alcohol) and Fatty Liver Disease, and (4) Type 2 Diabetes and Insulin Resistance (from your pancreas wearing out). Also, the fructose (from sugar) stimulates you to keep eating and eating (despite being full), and fatty acids exiting from the liver greatly encourage cancer cell growth! Plus, eating sugar reduces your immune system's defenses, and ages your brain more, to help cause early dementia and Alzheimer's disease!

These ten horrible side-effects of sugar cause your body to be run down, fatigued, diseased, and due for an early death. Indeed, sugar truly *is* the main toxic curse of our diet.

Thus, your drug-like "sugar high" just isn't worth it, especially when (instead) you can eat dates, raisins, bananas, all fruits and berries, dried fruits, (self-made) fruit juices, carob-flavored drinks, stevia (truvia), and milk sugar (lactose). Adding cinnamon can enhance any of these sweet tastes, too.

Incidentally, eating fruit is OK because of all the healthy micronutrients in fruit, plus lots of fiber. Also, the amount of fructose is relatively quite small, compared to the *enormous* amount of fructose in sugar!

Sum Up

(1) Our body has no need for the fructose-half of sugar.
(2) This fructose, like a toxin or poison, goes straight to the liver.
(3) Ten horrible side-effects result, including the possibility of dying earlier.
(4) We then feel rundown, fatigued, and diseased.
(5) So, we must stop sugar and instead eat fruit, dried fruit, fruit juices, stevia (truvia), carib, milk sugar (lactose), and cinnamon, for our "sweet-tooth" craving.
(6) The sugar that we stop must include white sugar, brown sugar, cane sugar, high-fructose corn syrup, honey, agave, maple syrup, molasses, aspartame (nutrasweet), saccharin (sweet 'n low), and sucralose (splenda), etc. which are all as bad as sugar.

When we've switched to the good sweets in (5), and stopped the bad sweets in (6), we'll feel healthier, live much longer, and lose weight to be much slimmer!

For 146 more reasons why sugar is bad for you, go to the blog post of Nancy Appleton, Ph.D, of September 2010 at http://www.sugarshock blog.com/index.html.

3

How I Stopped Sugar - My Story

When I read several books available from the internet on all the *bad side effects* of sugar, I realized that I needed to *stop sugar* (or else cut down). But I also realized that this would be nearly impossible, because I was such a *sugar addict* (to chocolate milk, ice cream, cookies, pies, chocolate bars, candy, soda pop, etc.)

Then, quite unexpectedly, I came across Anthony Shkreli's book *You Are Not Addicted, You Are Starving*, when it popped up by chance on my computer screen (after ordering some other book). What a miracle!

Anthony Shkreli's book contained dozens of pages explaining *how eating silica-rich foods stops your craving for sugar*! It's a bit complicated, but it can all be summed up as: (1) We're almost all of us silica-mineral deficient, (2) silica, as a needed nutrient, gives us numerous health benefits, and we *must* have it, (3) a small amount of silica is in sugar, due to how sugar is processed, (4) so, we *really* crave sugar because of the *silica* in sugar! (5) if we eat silica-rich foods, we'll get our silica from *foods*, instead of from sugar, (6) then our craving for sugar (which is really for the *silica* in sugar) will stop! (You might need to re-read this (1) to (6), to thoroughly understand it all.)

The nine best silica-rich foods are [numbers in mg silica per 100 g = 3.5 oz servings]: oats (595), millet (500), barley (233), organic potatoes with skin (200), sprouted whole-grain bread (158), rice, organic cucumbers with their skin, bell peppers, and organic turmeric powder. Silica is not "just another trace mineral", to continue to ignore.

I immediately began, that very day, eating lots of silica-rich foods. And, instantly, in just one day, all craving for sugar stopped! Incredible, right? So, I continued eating one of these nine silica-rich foods every day (for months now) and because there was no *craving* for sugar, I therefore *ate no sugar* at all for months! Amazing! Instant cold turkey! But I noticed that on days when I ate very little silica-rich foods, the sugar-craving immediately started up again. At these times, I would practically drool for ice cream or chocolate! To offset this sugar-craving quickly, I would immediately eat some sprouted, whole-grain bread, or cook up some oatmeal and quickly chew and swallow it down. Then, *presto!*, no more craving for sugar almost instantly.

Yes, the solution to stopping your sugar craving (by eating silica-rich foods) really works! But, you have to continue to eat silica-rich foods, every day. Of course, due to all the wonderful health benefits of silica (see chapter 4), you'll *want* to eat all these silica-rich foods anyway!

Note

Even though eating silica-rich foods stopped *my* sugar-craving, in just one day, others may require longer. Perhaps three or four days? A week? Two weeks? Obviously, some people will take longer than others for this method to work for *them*.

Incidentally, I did *not* have a very good experience, at all, with *silica supplements* (bought at a health food store, or online). I strongly recommend that you get your silica from *silica-rich foods*, and *not* from silica supplements (none of which worked for me).

The silica supplements—with just the inorganic mineral, dissolved in water, just coated the insides of my digestive tract and blood vessels—were *not* assimilated. The organic, chelated silica supplement were an extract from the *horsetail herb*, from which I got allergic side effects of nausea, exhaustion, and kidney pain.

But supplements of *powdered turmeric* work well to provide silica, since turmeric is a plant that strongly absorbs silica from the soil. Also, turmeric supplements are quite healthy for you in many other ways besides their very high silica content. So, taking supplements of organic powdered turmeric is highly recommended for your silica intake!

4

Numerous Silica Health Benefits

Silica is not "just another trace mineral" to continue to ignore. Instead, silica *very powerfully* promotes overall good health! Silica helps you to stay younger longer, and stops "early aging". Wounds heal much faster with silica. Bone and connective tissue, especially collagen, build more rapidly with silica. Silica helps to stop Alzheimer's disease, and prevents cardiovascular disease! Silica-rich foods and silica supplements revitalize your skin, hair, and nails, to make you look much younger, too!

Silica stimulates growth in bone fractures. Silica helps create healthy arteries. Silica helps the body to manage and balance water. Silica attracts many much-needed minerals. Silica balances pH. Silica greatly benefits the brain and cognitive behavior. Silica greatly reduces stress.

Obviously, all these incredible benefits mean that it *really makes sense* to eat plenty of silica-rich foods, to greatly enhance your overall good health (besides stopping your craving for sugar)!

5

Biggest Enemies Of Silica Absorption

These are the worst "stoppers" of absorbing silica:

1. *Aluminum*. Aluminum is toxic, and "pushes out" silica, so that the silica isn't absorbed! Try to reduce your intake of aluminum as much as possible. Don't use aluminum cooking pots, or drink soda pop from aluminum cans. Live in an area where airplanes aren't spraying "chem trails" of aluminum particles way up in the sky, which will eventually fall down (from high overhead) into your lungs and body, wrecking your silica absorption and health.

2. *Stress*. Reduce stress in your life as much as possible. Or even double your silica intake, to help you deal with all this stress.

3. *Sugar*, white bread, and refined grains, which practically do the *opposite* of silica, and cause many immediate and long term bad health problems. Cut down on them!

4. *Antibiotics*. These kill off your intestinal probiotics, so that vitamin B3 absorption is interfered with. Since vitamin B3 is a great *helper* of silica absorption, the wrecking of vitamin B3 absorption by antibiotics will greatly hurt silica absorption.

A "Silica Reserve" Is The Goal

Once you start silica ingestion, from silica-rich foods, your health and energy should gradually get better and better, until you've built up a "silica reserve", that you should try to maintain by continued daily silica ingestion. This "saturation with silica" is what will cause you to lose your craving for sugar, and be much healthier, mentally and physically.

6

Vitamin B3, In A Vitamin B Complex, Is A Big "Helper" To Silica

Vitamin B3 tremendously helps the assimilation of silica, and thus *could* be taken too, to speed up this whole process! But because the B-vitamins all work together as a "team", *all eleven* B-vitamins are *necessary* (in this remedy, to stop sugar craving). Vitamins B1 (thiamin), B2 (riboflavin), B3 (niacin or niacin-amide), choline (formerly B4), B5 (pantothenic acid), B6 (pyridoxine, pyridoxal, pyridoxamine), B7 (biotin), B8 (inositol), B9 (folic acid), B10 (PABA or para-aminobenzoic acid), B12 (cobalamins, such as cyanocobalamin) are all necessary, to be present , in the vitamin B complex. If even *one* of these 11 B-vitamins is missing, then find *another* brand of vitamin B complex, with *all these eleven* B-vitamins in it. This is very, very important! If you neglect this, and if even *one* B-vitamin is missing, then you'll gradually become deficient in the missing B-vitamin, and the whole remedy will be wrecked! I've found from experience that deficiency in the missing B-vitamin usually causes a type of "unexplained fatigue".

Also, the vitamin B3 in the B complex capsule needs to be vitamin B3 in the form of niacinamide and *not* niacin. This is because vitamin B3 as niacin causes an itchy, red, unpleasant flush in the face and all over the body. To prevent this extreme flushing irritation, vitamin B3 as niacinamide (and *not* niacin) should be taken. A good brand of multiple B vitamins, for only $7.99, is *Solaray B-Complex 50* in a 50 capsule bottle. It can be ordered at http://www.solaray.com, or by phoning 1 (800) 683-9640. Solaray B-complex 50 is highly recommended, since it has all the above requirements and is inexpensive!

Remember, though, that it's really silica that stops the sugar craving. Vitamin B3 (in a vitamin B complex) is just a "helper". But still, I highly recommend taking a vitamin B complex with the silica-rich foods!

7

Silica Is A Needed, Required Nutrient For Health

Even if you were not a sugar craver (and using silica to stop the sugar craving), you would still need plenty of silica for your health! Silica is such a needed nutrient, and all people living in our modern civilization are so *silica-deficient*, that it can confidently be said that silica ingestion can solve many of your problems resulting from this silica-deficiency! Thus, silica is the key to not only stopping sugar craving, but to building "super-health", which we all desire!

8

Final Thoughts

You have now finished this little book, that explains how the Silica System will stop your sugar craving. Also, I have told you just how to do it, with a few variations.

Now, the question is, are you going to do it? I really, really hope you do, and stop your sugar craving, and begin living a much healthier life!

But, people are very complicated psychologically, I've found, over many years. And often, at a point like this, people come up with all sorts of reasons and excuses *not* to do the thing next most indicated.

A "silver-tongued salesman" often walks in now, to "close the deal"! A stream of glib words, carefully chosen, to fill you up with extreme enthusiasm to try the Silica System (or some other kind of "sales abracadabra").

But the trouble is, I'm *not* any kind of salesman or promoter. Sorry! I *don't have* the "magic words" to transform you from a "reader" into a "Silica System Trier" (which will then result in your stopping craving sugar.)

So, I wonder if you'd do me a small favor. Could you bring onto the stage of your "inner psyche", *your own* Inner Salesman/Promoter? What would *your own* Salesman/Promoter say to you right now? What "wise words of wisdom" seem to come into your mind now, encouraging you to give the Silica System an honest try?

Perhaps Inwardly You Hear

(1) "Boy, this silica thing is interesting. I wonder if it works? If it does, it would be great! But if it doesn't, I am *so tired* of trying these "stop-sugar things" that don't work! But this "silica thing" only involves eating a few silica-rich foods every day. And silica-rich foods are good for me, anyway. Okay! Why don't I give silica-rich foods a try, for just *two weeks*, and see what happens?

Or perhaps inwardly you hear . . .

(2) Something else!

Obviously, every single person reading this short book is *unique*, and I have *no* idea what's going on inside you, now. Also, not being any kind of salesman, I have no idea what to *say* to you anyway, about what's going on within you, now.

But please, could you just *try* this Silica System? From my heart, I'd really like you to stop craving sugar and begin to live a more wonderful life! And then tell your friends, who will listen to you, so that they'll try the Silica System too, and then they will tell *their* friends!

I care about you, and I want very much for the Silica System to stop your sugar craving, if you truly want this, too.

Anyway, if it just so happens that you *do* try the Silica System for two weeks, I would really like to hear about your results, *whatever they are*. Please, send me your results to my email: garypickler1@gmail.com.

Thank you, thank you so much, for trying the Silica System, passing it on, and helping to heal more and more people from their sugar craving!

9

Other Ways To Stop Craving Sugar

(1) Eat "Raw Meal" (protein powder), flax oil, milled/ground up flax seeds, turmeric powder, and blue green algae. This remedy can be used for other sugar cravings, too. This *combination of super foods* (eaten whenever I craved ice cream) stopped my addiction to ice cream (before I discovered silica-rich foods).

(2) Nancy's brand *kefir* (only this brand, not any other) in many fruity flavors. This healthy substitute can be used for other sugar-drink cravings, too. By drinking Nancy's kefir, whenever I craved chocolate milk, I was able to stop my years-long addiction to drinking a quart of chocolate milk every day.

(3) Drink plenty of water. Most people don't drink enough water and live their life quite dehydrated. Try a glass of water instead of eating sugar when the sugar craving strikes.

(4) Get sufficient sleep. It may be that you're tired from insufficient sleep, and unknowingly using sugar as a "pick-me-up".

(5) Eat foods that are "healthy fat", instead, especially if they have Omega 3, 6 or 9 fatty acids. Eggs, nuts (without peanuts), nut butters, avocados, fish, etc.

(6) Organic food. It is healthier and gives you more energy, so that you won't need "sugary dessert" afterward.

(7) Eat fruit, dried fruit, or fruit juice (diluted with water) instead of a sugary treat.

(8) Use stevia instead of sugar.

www.ingramcontent.com/pod-product-compliance
Lightning Source LLC
Chambersburg PA
CBHW030105300526
45785CB00019B/2748